ANTIOXIDANTS

Remi Cooper

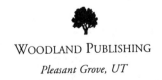

WOODLAND PUBLISHING

Pleasant Grove, UT

© 1997
Woodland Publishing
P.O. Box 160
Pleasant Grove, UT
84062

The information in this book is for educational purposes only and is not recommended as a means of diagnosing or treating an illness. All matters concerning physical and mental health should be supervised by a health practitioner knowledgeable in treating that particular condition. Neither the publisher nor author directly or indirectly dispense medical advice, nor do they prescribe any remedies or assume any responsibility for those who choose to treat themselves.

TABLE OF CONTENTS

ANTIOXIDANTS: AN INTRODUCTION

Antioxidants have been the subject of much research and writing in recent years. It has long been known that they fight the effects of free radicals and do much to slow down the aging process and prevent various types of disease. It has been established that more than sixty human diseases involve free radical damage, including cancer, heart disease and immune system decline. To better understand why a comprehensive antioxidant program is a key element of continuing good health, it is important to know how free radicals and oxygen affect our bodies, and what the various antioxidants are and how they work.

FREE RADICALS

Antioxidants are necessary because they fight the effects of free radicals in the body. Free radicals are molecules with electrons that are unpaired. If a molecule has an electron that does not have a partner, it becomes unstable and reactive. Free radicals steal electrons from other stable molecules in order to become stable themselves. Once the electrons are paired, the molecule becomes stable and nonreactive. When a stable molecule loses an electron to a free radical, it becomes another free radical that will in turn steal an electron from yet another molecule. And so a destructive cycle begins. Basically, "each time a molecule loses an electron, it is damaged and will damage another molecule."[1] Radicals do not react with any great selectivity, and the chain reactions they set off are a basic principle of free radical chemistry.[2]

It is true that when two free radicals meet, their unpaired electrons can join together to create a stable pair. This does not happen often, however, because most molecules present in living organisms do not have unpaired electrons. This means that any free radicals that are produced will most likely react with nonradicals, thus creating new free radicals.

Free radicals are formed as a result of normal body functions or the interaction of factors external to the body. As the body uses nutrients and oxygen to create energy, oxygen molecules with unpaired electrons—free radicals—are created. These by-products of normal metabolism cause extensive damage to DNA, protein and lipids. Exposure to radiation, whether from the sun or medical X-rays, and environmental pollutants such as tobacco smoke and car exhaust also contribute to the formation of free radicals.

It is important to understand that free radicals are not all bad. In fact, we need free radicals to live. They benefit the body by destroying alien bacteria and helping to fight off infection. They help with the constriction of blood vessels by influencing the tone of the tissue lining of the vessels. Free radicals are also important in producing vital hormones and activating certain enzymes.[3] The danger comes when excessive and uncontrolled amounts of free radicals are present in the body. Diet, exposure to toxins and radiation, exercise, illness, and certain medications increase oxygen-related reactions in the body and the number of free radicals increases.

Because oxygen is necessary for all body functions and is the cause of most free radical activity, it is necessary to understand how oxygen affects the body and how it contributes to free radical activity.

THE IMPORTANCE OF OXYGEN

The element oxygen (chemical symbol O) exists as a double molecule—two atoms being joined together to give O_2 (dioxygen). It is an odorless, tasteless, colorless gas. The percentage of oxygen in the air is approximately 21 percent, making it the second most abundant element in the atmosphere. Beyond the oxygen found in air, oxygen is also found in water (H_2O) and in mineral ores. Oxygen is by far the most common element in the earth's crust. Oxygen has limited solubility in water, which is crucial to the survival of fish and other water organisms, and essential for the respiratory functions of human beings. Oxygen has to dissolve in water to cross the alveoli of the lungs and reach the transport organisms of the blood.

Oxidation

A big problem with oxygen is that it *oxidizes* organic molecules, including foods, plastics, paints, fuels, rubber and human tissue. Basically what happens when a molecule is oxidized is that it is attacked by oxygen and forms an oxide. Common examples of oxidation are apple slices turning brown, oil going rancid, and machine metal rusting. The oxygen molecules that damage the apples, the oil and the metal are called oxidants. They oxidize other molecules by either taking hydrogen, adding oxygen, or taking electrons from them. In turn, oxidation often results in the formation of more oxidants, or free radicals.[4] It is these free radicals that break the body down, cell by cell, tissue by tissue, just like rust in the machine.

The rates at which oxidation occurs are very slow at normal temperatures. However, the rate of oxidation processes can be increased by enzymes or by heat. Antioxidants—substances that fight against oxidants that cause free radicals—prevent oxidation by removing catalysts. They also protect important cell components by being oxidized themselves or by repairing the damage caused by oxygen.

The irony is that even though molecular oxygen is absolutely required to produce the fuel which sustains cell life, it also presents a threat. O_2 (dioxygen) has two electrons, but it qualifies as a free radical because it contains two unpaired electrons. Under ideal conditions, oxygen is tightly coupled, as in H_2O (water), but this is not always the case, and oxygen is available as a free radical within the body.[5]

Oxygen Reduction

In biological systems, most attention has been focused on the oxygen radicals because they seem to be the most common and the most damaging. Here the discussion will focus on two important radicals—superoxide and hydroxyl—that result from the reduction of oxygen. Reduction is a process similar to oxidation that results in the production of free radicals. Reduction is done by adding electrons to a molecule, adding hydrogen, or by removing oxygen. The chemical that actually does the reduction is known as the reducing agent.[6] A simple example of reduction would be:

$$CO_2 + C \rightarrow 2CO$$

This equation would be read "carbon dioxide (CO_2) is reduced to carbon monoxide (CO) and carbon (C) is oxidized to carbon monoxide (CO)." With both processes at work, oxidation and reduction can change a carbon dioxide molecule and a carbon atom into two molecules of carbon monoxide. Another example can show how the addition of electrons through reduction can change the chemical make-up of an atom.

$$O_2 + e^- \rightarrow O_2^-$$

In this equation, oxygen is reduced to a free radical known as a superoxide radical.

Superoxide Radical

Superoxide is a radical made by adding one electron to an oxygen molecule (O_2). The added electron pairs with one of the unpaired oxygen electrons leaving one unpaired electron. The resulting radical can act as a weak oxidizing agent by accepting one more electron. For example, it can oxidize ascorbic acid (vitamin C). The chemical behavior of superoxide depends on what it is dissolved in. In water, it is not highly reactive, but in organic solvents it is far more reactive and dangerous. In fact, any superoxide produced within the body might do considerable damage.[6]

Hydroxyl Radical

The hydroxyl radical is the most reactive oxygen radical known to chemistry. It is extremely reactive and attacks whatever it comes in contact with. Hydroxyl will pull hydrogen atoms off whatever it can and convert itself back into water.[7] It is quite unselective in the damage it produces, and can set off various free radical chain reactions. The danger comes when hydroxyl radicals start pairing off with DNA constituents, preventing normal pairing and resulting in DNA mutations that cause such diseases as cancer.[8]

Singlet Oxygen

Although oxygen (O_2) has two unpaired electrons, these electrons are paired in such a way that O_2 oxidizes most things very slowly at room temperature. One theory of aging is that aging is caused by slow, cumulative oxidation of body tissue over time. Oxidation is accelerated by heat and catalysts, and with a simple change in its electron pattern, O_2 can convert into singlet oxygens, which are more powerful, more reactive oxidizing agents.[9] Singlet oyxgen quickly oxidizes lipids (fats) and changes them into lipid peroxides (see next section).

THE ROLE OF LIPIDS

In any discussion of free radicals and oxidation, it is important to discuss the role of lipids (fats). Oxidation—the creation of free radicals from oxygen—occurs more readily in fat molecules than it does in carbohydrate or protein molecules. Lipids are more susceptible to to free radical attacks because their electrons are held more loosely than those of other molecules.[10] Free radicals cause *lipid peroxidation* which, simply said, is destruction by free radicals. John M. Gutteridge of the Oxygen Chemistry Laboratory in London explains:

> Every body cell has a membrane that consists of a phospholipid bilayer. Proteins are embedded in this layer to perform specific functions, such as transport molecules and enzymes. To function properly, the membrane must be 'fluid' (i.e. its constituents must be able to move around freely). Fluidity is largely determined by the presence of polyunsaturated fatty acid side chains in the membrane lipids. The downside is that the polyunsaturated fatty acid side chains are very susceptible to free radical attack, which can start off lipid peroxidation. Peroxidation causes damage to membrane lipids and proteins, and depletion of antioxidants.[11]

Reactive free radicals (such as the hydroxyl radical and singlet oxygen) both contribute directly to peroxidation. They pull hydrogen atoms off polyunsaturated fatty acid side chains and those atoms bond with carbon molecules. As a result one of the carbon electrons is left unpaired—a free radical. These carbon radicals often combine with oxygen found in the cell membrane and form other highly reactive radicals.[12]

Protection of cell membranes from peroxidation and resulting free radical activity is achieved three ways: radical scavenging, lipid repair and lipid replacement. Antioxidants work to accomplish this. For example, vitamin E is the most powerful radical scavenger in cell membranes and glutathione peroxidase is an enzyme that helps repair damaged fatty acids.

THE MAJOR ANTIOXIDANTS

Antioxidants are the body's major defense against free radicals. Their name suggests that they work against those substances that create oxidants, the reactive substances that result from oxidation and reduction. Antioxidants fight free radicals by neutralizing them—they supply the missing electron and so stabilize the molecule. There are various types of antioxidants: dietary antioxidants and those that the body produces itself. The four major antioxidant nutrients are vitamin A (beta carotene), vitamin C, vitamin E and selenium. The antioxidant enzymes that the body produces to defend itself include glutathione peroxidase and superoxide dismutase.

Vitamin A

Vitamin A, the first vitamin to ever be isolated, is necessary for proper function of the eyes and for maintenance of the skin. Its scientific name is *retinol* because it is found in the retina of all mammals. It is also found in the liver, which stores about 90 percent of a healthy person's vitamin A.

Vitamin A works generally to bolster our resistance to infections. Carolyn Reuben, the author of *Antioxidants: Your Complete Guide*, explains that vitamin A works by keeping all the linings in the body healthy. It is essential for the health and moisture of the skin and the specialized cells lining the eyes, nose, mouth, throat, lungs, esophagus, stomach intestines, and urinary tract. These cells are the epithelial cells and when they don't have sufficient vitamin A, they thicken and harden. This is detrimental to health because, for example, "if the lining of the digestive or respiratory system is thickened and hard, it cannot pulsate well enough to move potentially harmful particles away from the lungs in either direction, and one becomes more susceptible to infection."[13] The skin and mucous membranes are our first line of defense against invading toxins and microorganisms, so we would do well to enhance its strength by supplementing our diet with vitamins such as vitamin A.

As it works to maintain the health of skin cells and mucous membranes, vitamin A protects the body from cardiovascular disease and cancer. This vitamin is necessary for new cell growth, which is important in slowing the aging process.

DOSAGE

A potential problem with vitamin A is that it can build up to toxic levels within the liver. This is not usually a problem, but to avoid the possibility, simply take beta carotene. The body converts beta carotene to vitamin A as needed, thereby averting the danger of toxic levels of the vitamin. Because vitamin A is a fat-soluble vitamin, it will not be absorbed on a no-fat diet. At least five grams of fat a day are necessary for adequate vitamin A absorption.

Beta Carotene

The compounds that form vitamin A are of two types: retinoids, or preformed vitamin A; and carotenoids, precursors of vitamin A that the body converts into active vitamin A.[14] Beta carotene is the best known of the carotenoids. It is actually composed of two vitamin A molecules that are split apart by liver enzymes when the body is low in vitamin A. If body levels are sufficient, however, the enzymes remain inactive and the beta carotene does not divide. For this reason beta carotene is considered a safe source of vitamin A and does not produce the toxic effects that come with high levels of vitamin A itself. If excess beta carotene is consumed, it is merely stored in fat tissue or may circulate in the blood.

Unlike vitamin A, which has limited antioxidant properties, beta carotene is one of the most powerful antioxidant nutrients. It can prevent free radical formation and inactivate existing free radicals. After free radicals have been formed, it traps them and breaks the chain reaction that they cause.

Beta carotene also absorbs and distributes energy from reactive forms of oxygen (singlet oxygen), thus making them more stable.[15] According to Richard Passwater, Ph.D., beta carotene may neutralize singlet oxygen before it can initiate skin and lung cancer. What makes beta carotene even more valuable is that—unlike vitamin E, which is destroyed in returning singlet oxygen to its natural state—beta carotene remains intact and can continue working against oxygen radicals.[16]

Beta carotene also works to destroy carcinogens (cancer-causing substances). Various studies illustrate its power against cancer. A study done in 1985 found that beta carotene, along with other carotenes that do not covert to vitamin A, protected the skin of animals from tumors caused by ultraviolet light and chemicals.[17] In another laboratory study, normal cells were injected with tumor-inducing agents or were treated with X-rays. Results confirmed that beta carotene can inhibit malignant transformation in normal cells.[18] Beta carotene has also been shown to be effective against cancer of the lungs, and to help protect the eyes against damage that may lead to cataracts.[19] In a 1992 survey of the impact of antioxidants on various cancers, researchers found that high levels of beta carotene in the blood were associated with a strikingly low incidence of cancer.[20]

Gaby and Singh, two nutritionists who have done much work with vitamins, offer an interesting insight into the value of beta carotene. It seems to do its best antioxidant work in areas of the body that have low concentrations of oxygen, such as capillary beds. Other antioxidants, like vitamins C and E, are more effective in more oxygen-rich environments. As a result, beta carotene's actions complement those of the other antioxidants.[21] For this reason, beta carotene and vitamin E should be taken together to receive the full benefits of each.

DOSAGE

A typical dosage of beta carotene is 25,000 I.U. This is the equivalent of eating about five large carrots daily. It can be taken at any time during the day.

Vitamin C

Vitamin C has an important role in various body processes necessary for life. Of key importance is its role in collagen formation. As nutritionist Gary Null explains, "Collagen is protein that works like glue to bind cells together to form tissues. The very structure of the body—the skin, bones, teeth, blood vessels, cartilage, tendons, and ligaments—depends on collagen. And the integrity of collagen, in turn, depends on vitamin C."[22]

Consequences of a lack of vitamin C were known long before its nutritional functions were known. The Egyptians, Greeks, and Romans, as well as Spanish, Portuguese, and English sailors were well aware of the lethal effects of scurvy, a disease in which collagen disintegrates within the body, leading to widespread internal bleeding and death. The British Royal Navy Physician Lind is actually credited with curing scurvy in 1753 by giving affected soldiers oranges and lemons.

The scientific name of vitamin C, *ascorbic acid,* actually means "without scurvy." Some scientists believe that cancer, atherosclerosis and other degenerative diseases are actually manifestations of mild scurvy. Although only about 60 mg of vitamin C is necessary to prevent scurvy, that may not be enough to provide optimal health. With time, a less-than-optimal intake of vitamin C can result in a mild deficiency of the nutrient and result in a person having increased susceptibility to many diseases.[23]

Vitamin C functions as a one of the most powerful free-radicals to prevent damage that contributes to aging and age-related diseases. Most importantly, it scavenges the superoxide radical, the hydroxyl radical, and singlet oxygen. Because it is an excellent source of electrons, vitamin C effectively deactivates these radicals.

David J. Lin, in his book *Free Radicals and Disease Prevention*, explains that because vitamin C is a water-soluble vitamin, it works in the watery areas of the body—the blood plasma, lung fluid, eye fluid, and between cells. Since most of the body (about 80 percent) is composed of water, vitamin C's antioxidant role is especially important because it can fight aqueous radicals before they have a chance to damage body lipids.[24] By preventing lipid peroxidation, it prevents the formation of dangerous free radicals.[25]

Vitamin C works against pollution and toxins that damage cells and cause mutations. In fact, it may reduce some food carcinogens to inactive products and may protect lung lining fluids against damage by air pollution.[26] For example, vitamin C inhibits the formation of highly carcinogenic nitrosamines by reacting with nitrite before it can convert into nitrosamines.

Vitamin C is also crucial for the immune system. Studies show that it enhances immune function in various ways. In one study, healthy adults received one gram of vitamin C intravenously and after one hour the movement of their white blood cells had increased significantly. In another study 260 patients with viral hepatitis took 300 gms of vitamin C daily for several weeks. Researchers concluded that vitamin C "exerts a remarkable immunomodulating action." In patients with nasal irritation and congestion, vitamin C reduced symptoms in three-fourths of the patients.[27] More beneficial effects of vitamin C are that it increases immunity to infectious diseases, may lower total cholesterol, and enhances the effect of vitamin E. It also promotes wound healing, growth, tissue repair and helps in the utilization of iron.[28] Although research regarding vitamin C and the prevention of colds is conflicting, many studies show that it can shorten the duration and lessen the intensity. Vitamin C has also been used to reduce the symptoms of asthma and allergies.

Since vitamin C levels in the blood and body decrease with age, elderly subjects who take vitamin C supplements are rewarded with enhanced immunity. Results of a recent study show that men who consume 300 mg of vitamin C daily through food and supplements have a 40 percent lower death rate from heart disease and other causes than men whose intake is less than 50 milligrams.[29]

DOSAGE

We cannot produce this vitamin in our body, so our essential requirement must be met entirely by diet and supplementation. A typical dosage of vitamin C is about 2000 mg. Because vitamin C is water soluble, it is easily eliminated from the body, so taking it at various times during the day is helpful. Some dieticians recommend taking 1000 mg with each meal to keep blood levels up. If you have an unhealthy diet or are at risk for cancer for any reason, you would do well to take 2000 mg three times a day.[30]

Be aware that excessive amounts of vitamin C can cause intestinal discomfort (gas and possible diarrhea) in some people. If this occurs, simply cut back. Dr. Robert Cathcart III, M.D., who has treated more than 12,000 patients with vitamin C for a wide variety of viral illnesses, says the sicker you are, the more vitamin C you can take. Diarrhea is the sign of your *optimal* dose, so when it occurs, simply decrease the amount you're taking by 10 percent until you feel better and then increase your dosage gradually. Your body tolerance will improve rapidly. When taking large amounts of vitamin C, you should also supplement with magnesium and other nutrients.[31]

Vitamin C has a synergistic relationship with other antioxidants such as vitamin E and glutathione peroxidase. This may be due to the involvement of vitamin C and glutathione in the regeneration of vitamin E after it has reacted with a free radical.[32] For this reason, the more vitamin C you take, the less vitamin E you need.

Vitamin E

Vitamin E works to prevent aging by prolonging the useful life of cells in the body. For example, it has been shown that the red blood cells of those who take vitamin E supplements age far less than do the red blood cells of people who take no supplements.[33] Vitamin E also works to protect vitamin C and vitamin A from free radical activity, thus keeping them potent.

One of vitamin E's most impressive abilities is that it can stop a wildly proliferating free radical chain reaction as it is happening. It also plays a crucial role in preventing the peroxidation of lipids. Since cell membranes are composed of lipids, it is important that they be protected. Once damage is done by peroxidation or oxidation, nutrients can no longer pass through the membrane properly. Too many nutrients may cause the cell to grow irregularly and too few nutrients will starve the cell and kill it. If too many cells are destroyed or damaged, the body cannot function properly and disease sets in. By protecting the cell membrane, vitamin E combats disease.[34]

Because vitamin E is a lipid-soluble vitamin, this means it functions in fatty areas of the body (like the cell membrane). Just as oils are prone to rancidity, so are the cell membranes and thus every cell of the body. If you squeeze a few drops of liquid vitamin E into a new bottle of cooking oil, it will prevent the oil from going rancid and increase the life of the oil. Inside your body, the vitamin is also needed as the amount of polyunsaturated fatty acids increases in the diet.[35] The reason is that the more unsaturated a fat is, the more susceptible it is to oxidation. Ingesting large amounts of unsaturated fats without extra vitamin E will quickly use up the body's supply of the vitamin.[36]

As it strengthens the cell membranes, vitamin E also assists in warding off free radical attack from the oxidative compounds found in smog, cigarette smoke and other toxic products. Researchers estimate that a single molecule of vitamin E can protect up to 1,000 membrane lipid molecules from peroxidation. This protection is intensified when vitamin C is present.[37] In its role as cell protector, vitamin E also inhibits cell damage that could lead to cancerous mutations. In this way it helps to prevent cancer.

Besides working to prevent cell damage and cancer, vitamin E is also important in reducing the risk of heart disease. In 1993 the results of two studies done at Harvard University proved what had long been suspected in the scientific community. One of the studies followed 87,000 female nurses for eight years. During that time subjects regularly filled out questionnaires about their lifestyle and diet. After adjusting for age and other variables, researchers found that the women who had they highest intake of vitamin E had a 36 percent lower risk of coronary disease than those with the lowest intake. The subjects with the highest levels of vitamin E took supplements and did so for at least two years to show the benefit of lower risk of heart disease.[38]

The second study followed 22,000 male physicians for four years. Researchers found that the men who consumed at least 100 I.U. for four years had a 40 percent less chance of heart diseases. This benefit occurred even when blood cholesterol levels did not change.[39]

Vitamin E deficiency has been shown to result in decreased size of lymphatic organs, the production of fewer T-cells, a weakened white blood cell function, and a reduction in resistance to infection. Studies looking at the results of elevated levels of vitamin E, on the other hand, show enhanced antibody response and improved white blood cell activity and immune response.[40] Such research emphasizes that supplementing with vitamin E can be only beneficial to the body.

DOSAGE

A typical dosage of vitamin E is 400 I.U. daily. A study done giving people various dosages of vitamin E (60, 200, 400, 800, or 12,000 I.U) showed that only subjects who took 400 I.U. or more of the vitamin daily experienced a decrease in the susceptibility of lipid peroxidation.[41]

For people over the age of forty, 400 I.U. twice daily is beneficial. As we age, body systems—including antioxidant functions—function less efficiently. Researchers at Tufts University Center on Aging show that vitamin E supplementation enhances immunity of the elderly.[42]

Synthetic forms of vitamin E are not as available to the body as natural forms. In fact, the body only absorbs a small portion of synthetic vitamin E. Natural forms of vitamin E also 36 percent more bioactive than synthetic forms.[43] You can ensure you are buying a natural form of vitamin E by simply reading the label. Natural vitamin E is D-alpha-tocopherol, while synthetic vitamin E is DL-alpha tocopherol. Just remember you do not want the DL form.

Selenium

Selenium is one of the ten essential trace minerals and is present in all tissues of the body. Selenium is best known for its role as an antioxidant and its function in fighting cancer. It is the main component of glutathione peroxidase, an enzyme that neutralizes free radicals within and between cells. In order for the body to be able to produce this enzyme, selenium is essential.

Selenium specifically protects the liver from damage and works to stop lipid peroxidation. It is known that the mineral is vital in maintaining the elasticity of body tissues, and perhaps by preventing the oxidation of fatty tissue it helps to keep tissue supple. By doing so, it helps combat effects of aging. With the proper amount of selenium, the skin is more healthy, muscle mass and tone are more easily maintained, and the heart is strengthened. Without selenium, the heart "collapses into a flat, flaccid sheet of tissue, devoid of fiber and muscle."[44]

Research has also found a solid relationship between selenium and cancer. Hundreds of studies give evidence of its effectiveness. As early as 1969, two physicians noted the inverse relationship between the incidence of cancer and the amount of selenium in patients' blood samples.[45] In a later study done with mice, dietary selenium was found to reduce the incidence of breast cancer due to a virus that the mice ingested with their mother's milk from 80-85 percent down to 10 percent. Even more amazing is that in the 10 percent of the mice that still experienced cancer, it appeared 50 percent later, the tumors were less malignant, and the animals' survival time was 50 percent longer.[47]

According to Richard Passwater, Ph.D., a doctor who has done much research on selenium,

Many different types of laboratory experiments have been conducted and they all show that selenium is protective against cancer. Tumor cells injected into animals grow when the animals are selenium-deficient, but do not survive in selenium-fortified animals. These animals are protected against both carcinogen-induced cancer and virus-induced cancer. The research has been examined by many scientists and is considered meaningful.[47]

Selenium works in tandem with vitamin E—in fact, they are so complementary that the level of each nutrient in our body will affect our need for the other. "The amount of selenium required in the diet is inversely related to the dietary level of vitamin E and the two nutrients have mutually sparing effects upon the biological needs for both."[48] Where vitamin E serves the body in the fatty areas of the cells, selenium destroys fat-soluble oxidants in the watery areas of the cells. Vitamin E enhances the effect of selenium, and selenium improves assimilation of vitamin E.[49]

People do not maintain healthy levels of selenium for two reasons: the foods they choose to eat are low in selenium and/or the selenium content of the soil in which their food is grown is low. If fertilizer containing selenium is added to the soil, one of the problems is easily solved. A change in diet can also be beneficial. Supplementation is also good and will only benefit the body.

DOSAGES

You have to be careful with how much selenium you take because too much can be toxic. A dosage of 50-200 mcg is recommended as a safe daily supplement, and more than 200 mg is not usually recommended. Selenomethionine, the form of selenium found in plants, is better absorbed than sodium selenite, the form usually found in supplements. Check your local health food store for the natural form. And for best antioxidant use, take it with vitamin E.

Pycnogenol

Pycnogenol is an antioxidant that consists of a highly bioavailable flavonoid called proanthocyanidin. This flavonoid is extracted from either pine bark or grape seed and both sources are virtually identical. Some researchers assert that pycnogenol is fifty times more potent than vitamin E and twenty times more potent than vitamin C.[50]

Because it is so powerful, pycnogenol neutralizes free radicals with great rapidity, thus allowing cells to regenerate. The resulting benefits are various. Pycnogenol combines with collagen and helps maintain and restore skin elasticity. It protects capillaries and so helps prevent varicose veins and bruising. Pycnogenol also functions as a natural anti-inflammatory and helps treat joint pain and injuries. Human trials have shown that the flavonoids of pycnogenol can prevent peripheral hemorrhage, swelling of legs due to water retention, diabetic retinopathy, and high blood pressure.[51]

Coenzyme Q-10

Coenzyme Q-10 (co Q-10) is a substance that resembles vitamin E and is known to have antioxidant powers. A coenzyme is a substance that combines with other coenzymes to produce complete enzymes. Coenzymes like co Q-10 are needed to speed up certain bodily processes and facilitate the production of energy.[52] High levels of co Q-10 are found in the heart and in the fatty tissues of cell membranes, just like vitamin E. As with other antioxidants, levels of co Q-10 decrease with age. Recent studies show that supplementing with co Q-10 can significantly reduce heart disease, hypertension, and enhance the immune system.[53] In clinically controlled tests with heart patients, it was shown that angina pectoris responds favorably to co Q-10. Likewise, when volunteers who did not exercise regularly took 60 mg of co Q-10 daily for two months, there was a surge in their ability to withstand vigorous exercise.[54]

Antioxidant Enzymes

The enzymes that we need are manufactured by our DNA. They act as catalysts to make possible the thousands of chemical reactions that fuel the body. Three enzymes in particular function in the body as free radical scavengers: glutathione peroxidase, superoxide dismutase, and catalase.

Glutathione peroxidase deactivates free radicals before they can damage cells. When a hydrogen peroxide free radical is formed, for example, glutathione will reduce it to water. This is very helpful because such radicals transform into the even more dangerous hydroxyl radical.[55] According to Jeffrey Bland, Ph.D., glutathione is the primary constituent of antioxidant defenses in the heart, lungs, liver and blood cells. But it does not work alone—it needs selenium to function efficiently. Glutathione is also known to work synergistically with vitamins C and A.[56] For the most part, glutathione is found in supplements that include other antioxidant nutrients and enzymes.

Superoxide dismutase and catalase function together to stop the creation of free radicals. Superoxide dismutase breaks the free radical chain reaction by changing superoxide radicals to hydrogen peroxide. In turn, catalase reduces hydrogen peroxide to hydrogen and water. In this way the superoxide radical is completely defeated.[57] Just like glutathione, these enzymes are also dependent on minerals. Copper and zinc are both required for their operation. The best source of superoxide dismutase and catalase is live food. Seed sprouts from sunflower seeds, lentils, mung beans, clover, and radishes are superior sources.

THE ANTIOXIDANT ADVANTAGE

Understanding the value of each individual antioxidant is important, but it is even more crucial to understand that antioxidants function most effectively when they are taken together. Just as vitamin E and selenium mutually enhance each other's actions, other antioxidants also work well together. In many of the studies done, an entire array of antioxidants is given to subjects. It would be impossible to determine which effects are due to which nutrient. Instead, they work as a whole to benefit the body.

For example, in a study reported in the British medical magazine *Lancet,* elderly subjects were given small doses of vitamin E, beta carotene, and some other vitamins and minerals for a one-year period. The subjects taking antioxidants suffered from half as many colds, flu outbreaks, and other infectious diseases in comparison with control groups given a placebo pill. Those who did get sick recovered twice as fast as the placebo subjects.[58]

Diet

Something else to consider is that, even as we supplement our diet with vitamins, minerals and other nutrients, we should also attempt to get as many of our antioxidants as possible from natural food sources. Eating fruits, vegetables and grains gives our bodies the complete nutrition and fiber necessary to keep healthy. A review of 172 studies shows a consistent relationship between the inadequate consumption of fruits and vegetables and increased incidence of cancer.[59] A more startling statistic is that the quarter of the U.S. population with the lowest dietary intake of fruits and vegetables has double the rate for most types of cancer (lung, larynx, oral cavity, esophagus, stomach, colon and rectum, bladder, pancreas, cervix and ovary) than the quarter of the population with the highest dietary intake. Only 9 percent of Americans eat the five servings daily of fruits and vegetables recommended by the National Cancer Institute. Remember that taking supplements does not replace the value of a good diet.[60]

Exercise

Regular exercise is crucial for optimal body functioning. Exercise does increase oxygen reactions that can lead to free radical production, so if you regularly do high-intensity exercise, you should take antioxidant supplements to protect yourself from danger. In a study done at the University of Washington School of Medicine in St. Louis, eleven young men were given 600 I.U. of vitamin E, 1000 mg of vitamin C, and 50,000 I.U. of beta carotene daily. Nine other men were given a placebo. At the beginning of the study, all the men ran on a treadmill for thirty-five minutes and the free radicals they produced were then measured. When they were tested again six months later, the subjects who had been taking antioxidants formed 17 to 36 percent fewer free radicals than those taking placebos.[61] In his book *Antioxidant Revolution,* Dr. Kenneth Cooper asserts that antioxidant supplements are *mandatory* for adults who exercise.[62]

CONCLUSION

Antioxidants are obviously an advantage against the aging process and against many diseases. Research shows that antioxidants help fight heart disease, cancer, atheroscerosis, arthritis, AIDS, cataracts, Alzheimer's, hypertension, multiple sclerosis and Parkinson's disease, and others. After years of research at the Gerontology Research Center, aging expert Richard G. Cutler concluded that the more antioxidants found in the body, the longer an individual's life will be.[63] In order to live a long and healthy life, antioxidants should be a staple of any nutritional program.

ENDNOTES

1. Lin, David J. 1993. *Free Radicals and Disease Prevention: What You Must Know.* New Canaan, CT: Keats Publishing, Inc., 11.
2. Gutteridge, John M. C. and Barry Halliwell. 1994. *Antioxidants in Nutrition, Health and Disease.* Oxford: Oxford University Press, 7.
3. Cooper, Kenneth H. 1994. *Dr. Kenneth Cooper's Antioxidant Revolution.* Nashville and Atlanta: Thomas Nelson Publishers, 23.
4. Reuben, Carolyn. 1995. *Antioxidants, Your Complete Guide.* Rocklin, CA: Prima Publishing, 3-4.
5. Gutteridge, John M. C. and Barry Halliwell. 1994. *Antioxidants in Nutrition, Health and Disease.* Oxford: Oxford University Press, 5.
6. Ibid, 8.
7. Pryor, William A. 1994. "Free radicals and lipid peroxidation: What they are and how they got that way," in *Natural Antioxidants in Human Health and Disease,* Balz Frei, ed. Boston, MA: Academic Press, 4.
8. Gutteridge, John M. C. and Barry Halliwell. 1994. *Antioxidants in Nutrition, Health and Disease.* Oxford: Oxford University Press, 10.
9. Ibid, 14.
10. Lin, David J. 1993. *Free Radicals and Disease Prevention: What You Must Know.* New Canaan, CT: Keats Publishing, Inc., 22.
11. Gutteridge, John M. C. and Barry Halliwell. 1994. *Antioxidants in Nutrition, Health and Disease.* Oxford: Oxford University Press, 49.
12. Ibid, 51.
13. Reuben, Carolyn. 1995. *Antioxidants, Your Complete Guide.* Rocklin, CA: Prima Publishing, 16.
14. Lieberman, Sheri, Ph.D. and Nancy Bruning. 1997. *The Real Vitamin and Mineral Book.* New York: Avery Publishing Group, 65.
15. Lin, David J. 1993. *Free Radicals and Disease Prevention: What You Must Know.* New Canaan, CT: Keats Publishing, Inc., 44.
16. Passwater, Richard A., Ph.D. 1985. *The Antioxidants.* New Canaan, CT: Keats Publishing, Inc., 18.
17. Kornhauser, A., et al. (1975). Effect of dietary carotenoids on lymphocyte responses to mitogens. Federal Proceedings 44, 544.
18. Krinsky, Norman I. 1994. "Carotenoids and cancer: Basic research studies," in *Natural Antioxidants in Human Health and Disease,* Balz Frei, ed. Boston, MA: Academic Press, 244.
19. Null, Gary and Martin Feldman, M.D. 1993. *Reverse the Aging Process Naturally.* New York: Villard, 147.
20. Cooper, Kenneth H. 1994. *Dr. Kenneth Cooper's Antioxidant Revolution.* Nashville and Atlanta: Thomas Nelson Publishers, 33.

21. Null, Gary and Martin Feldman, M.D. 1993. *Reverse the Aging Process Naturally.* New York: Villard, 21.
22. Ibid, 117.
23. Lin, David J. 1993. *Free Radicals and Disease Prevention: What You Must Know.* New Canaan, CT: Keats Publishing, Inc., 48.
24. Ibid, 48.
25. Weiner, Michael A. 1986. *Maximum Immunity.* Boston: Houghton Mifflin, 107.
26. Gutteridge, John M. C. and Barry Halliwell. 1994. *Antioxidants in Nutrition, Health and Disease.* Oxford: Oxford University Press, 59.
27. Null, Gary and Martin Feldman, M.D. 1993. *Reverse the Aging Process Naturally.* New York: Villard, 121.
28. Cooper, Kenneth H. 1994. *Dr. Kenneth Cooper's Antioxidant Revolution.* Nashville and Atlanta: Thomas Nelson Publishers, 213.
29. Lieberman, Sheri, Ph.D. and Nancy Bruning. 1997. *The Real Vitamin and Mineral Book.* New York: Avery Publishing Group, 122.
30. Weil, Andrew, M.D. 1990. *Natural Health, Natural Medicine.* Boston: Houghton Mifflin Co., 185.
31. Weiner, Michael A. 1986. *Maximum Immunity.* Boston: Houghton Mifflin, 173.
32. Knekt, Paul. 1994. "Vitamin E and cancer prevention," in *Natural Antioxidants in Human Health and Disease,* Balz Frei, ed. Boston, MA: Academic Press, 200.
33. Lieberman, Sheri, Ph.D. and Nancy Bruning. 1997. *The Real Vitamin and Mineral Book.* New York: Avery Publishing Group, 76.
34. Null, Gary and Martin Feldman, M.D. 1993. *Reverse the Aging Process Naturally.* New York: Villard, 134.
35. Reuben, Carolyn. 1995. *Antioxidants, Your Complete Guide.* Rocklin, CA: Prima Publishing, 40.
36. Lin, David J. 1993. *Free Radicals and Disease Prevention: What You Must Know.* New Canaan, CT: Keats Publishing, Inc., 53.
37. Null, Gary and Martin Feldman, M.D. 1993. *Reverse the Aging Process Naturally.* New York: Villard, 138.
38. Stampfer, Meir J., et al. 1993. "Vitamin E consumption and the risk of coronary disease in women," *New England Journal of Medicine,* 328, 1444.
39. Lieberman, Sheri, Ph.D. and Nancy Bruning. 1997. *The Real Vitamin and Mineral Book.* New York: Avery Publishing Group, 78.
40. Weiner, Michael A. 1986. *Maximum Immunity.* Boston: Houghton Mifflin, 109.
41. Null, Gary and Martin Feldman, M.D. 1993. *Reverse the Aging Process Naturally.* New York: Villard, 78.
42. Ibid, 135.
43. Lin, David J. 1993. *Free Radicals and Disease Prevention: What You Must Know.* New Canaan, CT: Keats Publishing, Inc., 54
44. Ibid, 56.
45. Passwater, Richard A., Ph.D. 1985. *The Antioxidants.* New Canaan, CT: Keats Publishing, Inc., 45.
46. Ibid, 45.

47. Ibid, 47.
48. Lonsdale, Derrick. 1986. "Free oxygen radicals and disease," *1986: A Year in Nutritional Medicine,* monograph. New Canaan, CN: Keats Publishing, Inc., 14.
49. Weintraub, Skye. 1997. *Selenium: The Health Connection.* Pleasant Grove, UT: Woodland Publishing, 24.
50. Elkins, Rita. 1995. *Pycnogenol: The Miracle Antioxidant.* Pleasant Grove, UT: Woodland Publishing, 13.
51. Lieberman, Sheri, Ph.D. and Nancy Bruning. 1997. *The Real Vitamin and Mineral Book.* New York: Avery Publishing Group, 200.
52. Reuben, Carolyn. 1995. *Antioxidants, Your Complete Guide.* Rocklin, CA: Prima Publishing, 53.
53. Ibid, 54.
54. Tenney, Deanne. 1996. *CoEnzyme Q10.* Pleasant Grove, UT: Woodland Publishing, 4.
55. Null, Gary and Martin Feldman, M.D. 1993. *Reverse the Aging Process Naturally.* New York: Villard, 158.
56. Ibid, 158.
57. Ibid, 160.
58. Cooper, Kenneth H. 1994. *Dr. Kenneth Cooper's Antioxidant Revolution.* Nashville and Atlanta: Thomas Nelson Publishers, 30.
59. *Natural Antioxidants in Human Health and Disease,* Balz Frei, ed. Boston, MA: Academic Press, xxiii.
60. Ibid, xxiv.
61. Cooper, Kenneth H. 1994. *Dr. Kenneth Cooper's Antioxidant Revolution.* Nashville and Atlanta: Thomas Nelson Publishers, 67.
62. Ibid, 70.
63. Ibid, 34.